MW00565997

The Answer!
By Phil Kaplan

It's Time This Whole Fitness and Weight Loss Thing
Started Making Sense.
The Time is Now!
The Answer is Here!

Including The Most Powerful Method
Of Shedding Fat and Transforming Your Body
In Seven Simple Steps!

"The Answer" is designed to "clear up" the misinformation that has prevented millions of Americans from living in bodies they love. The book is intended to be read and absorbed in 90 minutes and is not meant to prescribe specific programs or routines nor is it meant to substitute for personal consultation with a fitness professional. The information herein is presented in hope of allowing you to understand why your previous attempts at fitness might have left you frustrated and to empower you to find the changes you seek. It is protected by a Copyright 1999, Phil Kaplan. All Rights are Reserved. Reproduction without the written consent of the author is prohibited. For additional fitness services, Phil Kaplan can be reached at (954) 389-0280 or on the web at http://philkaplan.com.

The Answer
Copyright 1999, Philip A. Kaplan
P. A. Kaplan & Associates
a division of Personal & Club Development, Inc.
1304 SW 160th Ave., Suite #337
Fort Lauderdale, Florida, 33326

All rights reserved. No part of this publication may be reproduced or
transmitted in any form or by any means, electronic or mechanical, including
photocopy, recording, or any information storage and retrieval system
without the written permission of the publisher.

Distributed in U.S. by Personal Development, a division of Personal & Club
Development, Inc.
1304 SW 160th Ave., Suite #337
Fort Lauderdale, Florida 33326

Library of Congress Cataloging in Publication Data

Kaplan, Phil
        The Answer
        ISBN: 1-887463-17-8

To Order additional Phil Kaplan products call 1 800 552-1998
To reach Phil Kaplan's private offices call (954) 389-0280

Contents

Introduction

Lucy plowed through the supermarket. She was about to start her diet . . . again. After all, it had worked before! In fact, it worked five or six times before. She'd lost as much as thirty-eight pounds with "the diet." She spent last evening cleaning out her refrigerator, throwing away all of the "fattening stuff," and now she was buying all of the low fat, fat free, and healthy selections that were in the "OK" column on her diet list. She loaded her cart with those "good for you" low-calorie shakes, hit the low-cal snack section, and proceeded to the check-out line.

Oh no! Out of the corner of her eye, Lucy noticed that two lanes over, bubbly as ever, that perky little aerobic instructor from the Athletic Club was fidgeting, or dancing, or whatever it was that those obsessed aerobic people do. Little Aerobic Cindy waved and Lucy ignored her, at least for awhile. As Cindy became more and more animated, Lucy could no longer pretend that she didn't hear the *"hey, Luuuuucy"* screams echoing through the checkout area. She forced a smile and waved.

"I haven't seen you in class! What happened to you?"

Lucy knew that would be the first question out of that irksome little bundle of energy who had no idea what it was like to have the sluggish metabolism of a sleepy turtle. She only hesitated for a moment before coming up with, *"Oh, I've been so busy. I just haven't had time."* Sure it was an excuse, but Lucy wasn't about to tell the truth. The fact that no matter how hard Lucy jumped around and sweated, the only thing that worked for her was "the diet." Exercise just wasn't for her. Little size-one Cindy would never understand.

As Cindy danced her one-hundred-ten pound body closer, her eyes scanned Lucy's items. *"Are those weight loss shakes?"* Lucy wished a big gust of wind would come blow this annoying little nuisance off into aerobic land. *"Are you going back on that diet? Didn't I tell you a hundred times?"*

"No," Lucy thought silently. *"You told me in that squeaky voice a thousand times and if I hear it again I'm gonna lose my healthy breakfast all over your new aerobic shoes!"* Of course those words remained in her mind as she just tried harder to force a half smile and muttered something like, *"Uh-huh."*

"Stop going on diets! All you have to do is . . . . EAT RIGHT AND EXER-CISE!!!!!"

Thankfully the cashier blared out, *"next,"* and Lucy could now pay for her diet foods, get out of the store, and be free of that little aerobic pest. This time the diet *will* work . . . and she'll keep the weight off. Yeah, this time it will be forever! She doesn't need ice cream in her life any way. And who needs pizza. She can live on rice cakes, fat free stuff, and shakes. Yeah, she'll soon be fit and she'll never have to listen to an obnoxious little fitness person again!

I believe we all know the outcome of this story. Lucy gets fat and blames herself! Is that a cynical prediction? No! It's a guarantee! It's inevitable!

Is Lucy doomed to a life of flab? Does she need to buy one of those books about just accepting yourself the way you are? Not if she finds *the Answer!*

If you know someone like Lucy, or anyone who has struggled with attempts at changing their body . . . you're about to become enlightened! Set aside time to read this book, a time when you will be uninterrupted. Read it carefully and understand each point before you go on to the next. With the Seven Simple Steps that you're about to explore you'll acquire the power to change! 90 minutes from now, that power will be yours!

Eat right and exercise. Many, just like Lucy, have learned to hate the words. If it were really that simple, this would be the shortest book ever written. Four words between two covers. You can see that there are more than four words on this page alone, so obviously there's a bit more to fitness mastery than, *"Eat Right and Exercise."* That doesn't mean, however, that the fitness buff who shares those words with you with the best of intentions is wrong. Those four words are the foundation of *The Answer* as well as the foundation of any true technology of positive physical change.

Too many fitness professionals, although well intentioned, are misdirected and are unprepared to educate those who are not gifted with a passion for exercise or the perception of a metabolic advantage. I know. I speak before the industry's most motivated health club owners and personal trainers at conventions and seminars. They're frustrated. They know "eat right and exercise" works. They're fully aware of the foundation. Why can't their clients, the members of their health clubs, and the rest of America and the world "just do it?" Many frustrated fitness professionals have not been taught to recognize that "the rest of the world," is caught up in a maze of misinformation. In order to undo the damage that failed attempts and fraudulent offerings have wrought, in order to truly bring results, it's important to see how each failed attempt at "eating right and exercising" destroys motivation, cannibalizes hope, and moves each discouraged attempter farther away from ever believing they can make use of this powerful foundation. In order for that foundation to support results, there are a number of challenges that must be dealt with.

The first challenge lies in understanding what "Eat Right." means. While tens of thousands of fitness-wanting Americans carefully measure calories and scan the supermarket shelves for the "healthiest" choices, many are inadvertently destroying metabolisms and preparing their bodies to become quite efficient at storing fat!

The second challenge lies in understanding that while exercise is healthful, without several vital factors in place, an all out "exercise attack" might backfire if it is viewed as the plan for achieving a lean, toned, healthy body. If you exercise without results, or even worse, if you exercise and find yourself moving in the wrong direction, it won't be long before you run from the thought of putting on exercise clothing or running shoes. Have you been there? I'm not surprised.

At the conclusion of every seminar I conduct, a cluster of people wait to thank me for helping them finally take control of bodies that had moved away from the visions they had of their physical ideals. Almost every one of the expressions of gratitude is accompanied by the words, *"Phil, you make so much sense."* At first I was amused by that. After all, why were they thanking me for making sense? Isn't that what I'm supposed to do? With time I came to understand that the only reason people are failing to live in bodies they are truly thrilled with lies in the fact that they are fostering some false information. They are being misled. At some time they adopted a single piece of bad information or a set of false beliefs, and these beliefs acted as mines along the road to optimal health and leanness. The road without the power of understanding is a rocky one at best. With the Answer as your guidebook, that road will soon become so smooth you'll glide along it as you find ongoing improvement in the way you look and feel. The true power to change lies in understanding, and the more these people searched for understanding, the more confused they became. After helping thousands transform their bodies, I began to understand the relief that came with understanding. After years of carrying around the burden of believing they were stuck in bodies that wouldn't respond, the "sense" that finally helped them find the "a-ha," the missing piece of the puzzle, the reason behind the failure to achieve results, sparked the true power to achieve.

Tell me I make sense and I'm now flattered rather than amused. I'm thankful that I have the opportunity to "make sense" for so many people, to provide them with "the Answer."

My appreciation of my power to reach people stops there. I usually leave a seminar feeling a short term sense of fulfillment, one that is quickly overshadowed by an acute awareness of my limitation. For every one that I reach, another five thousand are falling for fraudulent and often dangerous "solutions" to their fitness and body shaping challenges. To prevent myself from running off on a tangent, from letting my frustration with the state of the fitness and weight loss industries get the best of me, I'll save a very abbreviated glimpse at my story (someday a TV miniseries!) for the end of this book. For now I want you to realize two things:

1. You hold in your hands the true technology of physical change and in that lies the power to reshape your body virtually any way you want to. It takes a level of desire and determination to sort through all of the nonsense on the market promising you "miracles." In obtaining this book you've displayed that determination. For that I commend you.

2. My personal mission is to educate America so everyone can change, and in bringing you *the Answer*, I'm one step closer to overcoming my personal frustration and achieving my mission. For that I thank you.

The Answer

I know you want *The Answer* NOW! You don't want to read through pages and pages. My intention is to keep this book brief, to "make sense" so that you become empowered, and to allow you enough understandable and usable information so you can take control of your body immediately. I'll provide the complete Overview first, and then in the following pages I'll expand on this simple model for achieving physical excellence. I'll present the Overview right now and appropriately title it, Seven Simple Steps To Transformation!

The Seven Steps:
1. Know and Take Control of Your Metabolism
2. Eat Supportive Meals Frequently
3. Limit Fat But Recognize and Avoid Sugar
4. Don't Be Fooled by Labels and Hype –
   Buy and Eat Supportive Food!
5. Exercise Aerobically, but in Moderation
6. Challenge and Protect Muscle!
7. Change the Focus of Your Exercise Regularly
   For Ongoing Progress

By understanding and applying the power contained in those seven simple sentences you'll find you can literally shape your body as a sculptor shapes clay. You'll also find these Steps can take you far beyond a "look," far beyond a happy reflection in the mirror. They can offer you a lifetime of health, energy, and vitality you might never have thought possible.

QUESTION: *Why Doesn't Everyone Know These Seven Steps?*

There are a number of reasons the technology I'm sharing with you, although it works 100% of the time, has remained so elusive. Firstly, Americans have been so wrapped up in the quick fix syndrome, they're led to believe they can have anything in an instant. Doctors clever enough to cash in with sophisticated versions of scalpels and suction pumps are promising they can suck the fat away and give you the body you want. Pharmaceutical developers spend a fortune in getting the FDA to approve new "diet drugs" so that as soon as the side effects of one materialize in the public eye, a new one can jump in as the new money maker. Food labelers have learned to manipulate labeling laws so that they can capitalize on the American want for better nutrition without actually having to deliver what the labels promise. Degreed nutritionists are graduating colleges accumulating information from textbooks that relay "nutritional science" that's more than a decade old, much of it formulated by food sellers. I meet a great many overweight nutritionists. Hundreds have gone through my Body Transformation Program and finally filled in the missing pieces of the puzzle to take control of their own bodies and their own metabolisms. It all boils down to misinformation. America has become confused.

In March of 1998 I was privileged to meet Dr. Clifford Carlson. Dr. Carlson was probably near the 500th physician I'd met with in reference to self-application of *the Simple Steps*. He found me on the internet after searching for *the answer* to his health and fitness concerns. His search was actually in hope of preserving a life. His own. He had gone on one of these "new miracle" give-up-carbohydrates-and-lose-weight diets. Sure, he lost weight, but aside from suffering some mild annoyances ranging from dizziness to an inability to concentrate, a loss of lean body mass, and a metabolic slowdown, he found himself in the hospital with heart failure! After finding my Body Transformation Program, Dr. Carlson turned it all around and took control of his body for the first time in his life! Keep in mind, he had only good intentions. He wanted to find self improvement, and was victimized by the array and availability of misinformation . . . . and he's a doctor! So, if you can't turn to your doctor, if the textbooks are outdated, if product manufacturers control and manipulate information, is it any wonder the true technology has remained a mystery?

What Is The Body Transformation Program?

I've taken *the Seven Simple Steps* and systemized them so anyone, and I do mean anyone, can follow the path to finding physical excellence. I'm flattered by the accolades I've received for *the Program* and am often amused when it's referred to as revolutionary. The only thing revolutionary about it is the fact that it's the plain and simple truth! With that truth comes true power. Not confusion, but clarity. Not frustration, but achievement. The fact that such a program is considered revolutionary simply reveals the state of the industry today.

I guess another reason the *"revolutionary"* word has been applied so often is because my Body Transformation Program challenges convention. Keep in mind, however, that convention isn't working! Here are a few of the features of the Program that have people stunned, amazed, and ultimately thrilled:

Regardless of your present exercise time investment, you begin with only 12 minutes of moderate aerobic exercise per day. 12 minutes! That's it!

You lose fat eating what most people perceive to be a tremendous amount of food. In fact, a great many people wind up eating more than twice as much food as they had eaten prior and losing fat at a rate they describe as incredible!

There is absolutely no deprivation. I encourage, or better yet, I insist that everyone who follows the program pick one day a week, "the Cheat Day," and on that day eat literally anything! Nothing is off limits! Most people are shocked that they can embark on an ongoing path of achievement without ever giving up pizza, ice cream, or their favorite indulgences.

I can not, nor do I hope to give you *"the Program"* in this book. *The Body Transformation Program* takes you through 17 weeks and includes 9 hours of me on video and audio tape in addition to recipes, a journal, and hundreds of pages of reference material. Keep in mind, the Program is available, and I encourage you to consider obtaining the complete program, however, with The Answer, you'll come to understand the technology that makes my *Body Transformation Program* so effective.

In *The Answer* you'll find the foundation. While *the Body Transformation Program* asks you to invest hours in application and understanding, the information I'm compiling for you in this book should be in your head in its entirety in 90 minutes! If I can get you to understand this technology in less time than it takes to watch a movie . . . perhaps I really have done something revolutionary. The clock is ticking. Let's get right to *the Seven Simple Steps*, one step at a time.

Simple Step #1: Know and Take Control of Your Metabolism

Metabolism. We all know the word. When, however, I ask somebody to define it, they usually fumble for a concise definition and wind up giving an example of somebody they know who can eat anything and not get fat. Of course they "hate" that person for it. The examples usually run something like this:

> *"Well, there's this girl Nancy at work, and she just pigs out on donuts and milk shakes, and when we all go out for lunch, she eats a cheeseburger and fries, and . . . that rotten little runt weighs 100 pounds soaking wet! It's not fair! We can't stand her!!!"*

Before you start throwing darts at tiny Nancy's picture, know this:

You Are Not A Victim of Your Metabolism.
You Are Its Creator!

Pretty powerful if it's true! Well . . . it's true! You can take total control of your metabolism, without drugs, without absurd potions, and best of all . . . without ever going on a diet again!

Metabolism, by definition, very simply put, is the speed with which your body processes food. That's it! Knowing that people with weight challenges envy those with fast metabolisms should allow you the first bit of insight into recognizing that a diet, or the deprivation of food, can not possibly train your body to get better at burning through your meals!

Food, Calories, and Metabolism

Another word that everyone knows but few truly understand is the word, *calorie*. *"It's . . . ummm . . . . the food thing."* Actually, a calorie is a measure of heat. One calorie, more accurately referred to as a kilocalorie, is the amount of heat required to raise one kilogram of water one degree Celsius. What in the world does that have to do with food?

Well, at this very moment your body is producing heat. You know that under "normal" conditions, you are maintaining a body temperature near 98.6 degrees. In fact, every time you move, more heat production is required, thus a "calorie," while being a measure of heat, is actually a measure of fuel.

Old, outdated, nonsensical *diet wisdom* (a contradiction in terms) leads us to believe that all calories are created equal. At the risk of overstating the obvious, I'll pose this tell-all question, "if you were to consume 1000 calories every single day obtained solely from ice cream sundaes, would your body look and feel different than it would if you consumed 1000 calories per day coming from well balanced meals?"

The answer is obvious. Why, though, if calories are equal in measure, should they affect the body differently?

Remember, when you move, you increase heat production. Also realize that every bodily function that requires the expenditure of energy is going to require heat production. When you blink your eye, do you burn calories? Of course! Am I recommending rapid blinking to lose weight? Of course not. I can see it now. *"Hardly any effort. $25 per month. Come to our new rapid blinking center for weight loss."* Absurd? Sure. With an understanding of the truth, you'll start to recognize how absurd so many of the advertised "metabolic solutions" truly are. Obviously the caloric burn of an eye blink is minuscule. Recognize, however, that any movement requires heat and thus calories. When you digest food, do you burn calories? Yup! Different foods, however, require varying amounts of energy production for the act of digestion.

I've come up with the term "Supportive Nutrition" to define the intake of meals that support a metabolic boost. Let me introduce you to Joanne the Calorie Nut, and then, as we move toward Simple Step #2, I'll explain why some meals may be more supportive than others.

Joanne the Calorie Nut
Joanne came into my office with papers. Lots of 'em. She had written down her intake for a week. Oddly enough, she didn't speak in food terms as most people would. She spoke in numbers and categories. She didn't tell me that she ate chicken, but rather described eating "a 100 calorie serving" from her "meat group." Joanne spent so much time counting, weighing, and measuring, I'd have to believe she took all of the pleasure out of eating. She learned her diet science well. She knew that if she had some fat free yogurt in the afternoon, she'd have to skip the evening snack allowance. She knew that if she had croutons in her salad, she was going to have to sacrifice the "bread group" from her dinner. Joanne explained that when she started dieting she lost weight on 1200 calories a day. She also explained that she no longer "diets" but now lives a lifestyle which is made up of bizarre categories and numbers. She also explained that she now alternates between her 1200 calorie maintenance, and an 800 calorie "weight loss" phase. Yeah, Joanne

had this diet stuff down pat, except for one small detail. She came to me for a consultation . . . because she was FAT!!!! Now hold on, I don't say that to be rude. I say that because that's what she told me! *"Phil, I know how to diet, but . . . I'm fat!"* Never did Joanne question the method she was using. She didn't want to accept the plain evidence that the 1200 calorie diet that used to be a "weight loss" diet was now her "maintenance." In that simple revelation is plain and sheer proof that her metabolism is moving in the wrong direction. She had it boiled down to bad genetics. Joanne, sadly to say, is *not* a success story of mine. She's one that I lost. She refused to accept that her nutrition program might be flawed. She just wanted me to give her an exercise program. I refused. Exercise plus Starvation is going to equal a further destruction of metabolism. I'm hoping the day comes that Joanne accepts the truth. Until then she'll continue to weigh, measure, and starve, and find greater and greater dissatisfaction with her body. I share this story to point out how ludicrous the literal brainwashing of Americans into buying a completely ineffective method of weight loss has become.

Simple Step #1 involves understanding. Had Joanne been open to understanding metabolism, she could then begin to take control. I don't blame her. I blame the diet industry that destroyed her. Forget completely the idea of "counting calories." Rather than counting them, I'll help you to understand them and then I'll teach you to teach your body to literally determine its own calorie need. There is an innate intelligence within your body that I'll help you to tap into, and within a short period of time you'll learn to "listen" and your body will "tell" you just how to feed it! You'll learn to understand that beneficial thing you might have mistakenly thought to be a hindrance . . . your appetite!

Exercise, Muscle, and Metabolism

We will get back into calories and heat in a moment, but let's first understand the essence of that mystical thing called metabolism. Muscle is Metabolism. Muscle is actually the part of your body that initiates movement, thus muscle is the part of your body that burns calories. Remember, you are producing "heat," thus burning calories, at any given moment. Since muscle is the source of the heat production, you'll conclude that the more muscle you have on your body, the more calories you will burn. This applies not only during exercise related activity, but during sitting, driving, talking, having sex, thinking, clicking the little buttons on the remote control, and yes, even while sleeping! Does that mean you should seek out Herculean muscles? Not unless you want to look like Hercules. It does, however, illustrate the value of holding on to the muscle you have if you don't want your metabolism to slow down!

Quick Time Out For Another Story.

Debbie The Muscle Chick.
A good portion of my career was spent developing and operating fitness facilities. I was involved in opening a new athletic club which was part of an exciting new real estate development in South Florida. At the Grand Opening, we wanted to do everything possible to make it festive, fun, and entertaining. We had a few pro football players signing autographs. We arranged for aerobic exhibitions, music, food, and . . . a bodybuilding display. First the man went. He was a regional competitor who wowed the audience with his muscularity and his posing routine. Then, Debbie, a female accomplished competitive bodybuilder took center stage. Debbie was certainly far more muscular than your typical female athlete, and while she was a champion in bodybuilding circles, the crowd that day was in shock! While they "wowed" the male, they stared open mouthed at the woman with the huge biceps and massive back muscles. That's when I overheard the comment from a woman in the audience . . . *"Gross. She lifts weights. I never want to look like that. I'll do aerobics. I don't want to ever be like that muscle chick."*

Shortly you'll understand the flaw in that response. I did want to take this moment to point out, however, that women are often misled into thinking of muscle as masculine. Go back and read my description of muscle. Movement. Heat production. Metabolism. You must, and I emphasize must, protect the muscle you have if you are going to rid your body of fat effectively, and if you add even a bit, your metabolism becomes even faster! You do not just "turn into" Debbie the Muscle Chick. Joanne was quite apparently sacrificing muscle and in that her metabolism was getting slower and slower. Please, even if you are a woman who believes your only goal is weight loss, accept the fact that muscle plays a vital role in the fat burning process. Muscle is the only site where fat is burned. Lose muscle and you have reduced the size of your fat burning machine! I believe you get my point, but even if you don't, I'll remind you when we get into the Steps regarding exercise.

The Diet Trick

OK, getting back to food, let's get rid of the idea of deprivation as a solution once and for all. Whether it's disguised under the heading of sensible eating, or it proudly proclaims itself to be the New Miracle Diet, if it involves a deprivation of nutrients that the body needs to sustain metabolism, you will lose weight at your metabolism's expense. There is one guaranteed outcome that comes along with any diet. Long term fat accumulation!

Food is Fuel, Calories are Heat , and Some Foods Are "Hotter" Than Others! We've established that there is a difference between ice cream calories and "well-balanced meal" calories. I'll help you to understand a major reason for that difference and further help you to understand food and its relationship with your metabolism. That will ease us very nicely into taking on Simple Step #2.

Remember, anything that requires energy requires heat production and a caloric expenditure. Well, when you chew, swallow, assimilate, and digest food, that in itself is going to require calories. When you eat fat, your body doesn't have all that much work to do. Envision a glob of oil floating in water simply dividing in half. That fat division didn't appear to require much effort. When the fat that you eat gets into your digestive tract, it is very simply divided into smaller molecules, broken down into fatty acids, and either stored as fat or burned as energy. That's it! It's easy! To digestively "deal with" fat, therefore, does not require all that much energy. There's something else you should know. Many people count fat grams, but haven't a clue as to what a gram is. They may look at a label and note that a food has 2 grams of fat and 2 grams of protein, thus assuming it has an equal amount of fat and protein. The catch is, 1 gram of fat yields 9 calories and 1 gram of protein or carbohydrate only yields 4! That would mean a food with 2 grams of fat yields 18 fat calories, and if it had an equal number of grams of protein, those 2 grams would only equate to 8 calories. Calorically, therefore, that food would have more than twice as much fat as protein!

Now that you understand that, you'll understand that fat has more than twice as many calories as an equal amount (in terms of grams) of protein or carbohydrate. Since, however, fat is so simple for your body to process, it only requires about 5 calories of energy to digest and assimilate 100 calories of fat. Let's call that a 5% metabolic boost (5 calories out of 100 are burned as fuel).

Stop here and read the last paragraph again. (only once, then go on . . . otherwise you'll never make it past this point in the book!) I want you to understand the "food burns calories" concept completely. I want you to grasp the differences in "calories required" to "burn" the different nutrients. I'm going to encourage you to eat, and I want to make sure you completely understand why.

Now, a look at carbs. When you eat complex carbohydrates, your body has to produce enzymes to break apart that food into chains of sugars, slowly break apart the chains, and then produce insulin to transport those sugars through the wall of the digestive tract. That's only the beginning. That sugar then has to be stored as glycogen in the muscles or in the liver. Obviously, there's far more work involved than there is in metabolically processing fat. For every 100 calories of complex carbohydrate that you eat, your energy requirement will be approximately 10 calories, offering twice the metabolic boost of fat! If you substitute complex carbs for some of the dietary fats you may be ingesting, less than half the calories go in, and twice the calories are burned! Is this starting to "make sense?" If so, let's go on.

I also mentioned protein. Proteins are made up of amino acids all assembled in clusters of 22. Those amino acid clusters are broken apart into chains of two and three. Those chains, called di and tripeptides, are transported through the wall of the intestine, and then those chains are rebuilt to create or repair tissue. That's a lot of work! In fact, it might offer more than twice the calorie expenditure of carbohydrates. When you ingest 100 protein calories, you're going to expend 20-25 calories just to handle digestion!

It's pretty clear to see why there's more to the puzzle than simply measuring grams or counting calories. At least I hope it's becoming clear to you. If I stepped over the line and became just a bit too scientific, don't worry. I'll simplify this and make certain you fully understand.

- Fats are high in calories and provide very little metabolic benefit.
- Complex carbs are lower in calories and provide far more metabolic benefit than fats.
- Proteins may provide more than twice the metabolic benefit of complex carbs!

You do need all the macronutrients (proteins, fats, and carbs), but a new understanding of how calories relate to energy should help you understand that there is a definite metabolic advantage to eating (not starving!) if you structure the meals in such a way that they offer a benefit to the metabolism you are beginning to learn you have control over.

- If you embark on a deprivation diet or starve yourself metabolism slows.
- Support metabolism nutritionally and you burn more calories as a result of eating!
- Metabolism is supported by having a concern for muscle and learning to fuel your body supportively.

Take a breath.

Aaaaah. That feels good.

Know you're one step closer. You're becoming empowered!

You're learning.

I'm making sense.

Smile. It burns calories!

OK. Now we can forge on ahead.

Simple Step #2: Eat Supportive Meals Frequently

Remember, metabolism is the speed with which your body burns through food. Dieting or simply avoiding food is going to cripple metabolism. If you want to get your body good at burning through food, a vital step is to put food into the calorie burning machine frequently!

I know the fear that comes along with this idea if you've been through diet after diet convincing yourself that the diets worked but you failed. You're afraid that if you eat more food, you'll add weight! Well, guess what! Initially, if you step on the scale shortly after embarking on a supportive nutrition program, you might see the number going up. If, however, you understand why, you'll be thrilled!

Muscle is good. You know that. The scale can't differentiate between muscle, bone, water, clothing, fat, or your internal organs. The scale simply sums it all up and gives you a grand total. You already know that if you lose weight, but that weight is primarily muscle, your weight loss will be short-lived and anything but healthful. The real trick here is to hold on to muscle, bone, and the other good stuff while you rid your body of fat. When you are living in a body that held onto the good stuff, released and incinerated fat, and sped metabolism in the process, you have and maintain total control!

If you haven't been eating in what I've learned to call a "supportive" manner, and you suddenly switch over to taking in the right combination of proteins, carbs, and a small amount of essential fats frequently throughout the day, the muscles have greater fuel than they've had previously. Remember when I was discussing the caloric value of carbohydrates, I explained that glycogen is stored in the muscles? Well, glycogen is "muscle fuel." With greater complex carbohydrate intake, there is more "fuel" for the "fuel tank." When the muscles attract more glycogen, your energy reserves are increased. Glycogen attracts water. In fact, for every gram of glycogen that you hold in muscle, you will likely attract 2.4 grams of water. Muscle is primarily water, and while water retention in other parts of the body may be viewed as negative, if a muscle is holding more water, you have more muscle! No, men don't suddenly rip through their clothes like the incredible Hulk, and women don't turn into "muscle chicks." Eat supportively and you simply begin to develop a stronger metabolism with more fuel for the machine. If you step on the scale, you might see an initial weight increase. Since, however, muscle is our fat burning engine, that weight offers you a distinct fat burning advantage.

If seeing the number rise at times on the scale is going to distress you, I will not tell you this is not for you. It is! I'll just tell you to stay off of the scale!

Of course, as your body releases and burns fat, if weight loss is a goal, the pounds will vanish, but you must accept that in order for it to be permanent, it's going to be gradual. Get excited in knowing that when you do it right, the fat you lose is not coming back. Rather than trusting that obnoxious little scale to give you a number you'll like on a daily basis, smash the thing to pieces! Use the mirror and your clothing as gauges of your progress. As fat goes away, your clothing fits better. As fat goes away, you begin to appreciate the shape of your body. As fat goes away, you realize you are, perhaps for the first time in your life, in control of your metabolism.

The nutritional plan that allows your body to hormonally release fat on an ongoing basis, and to produce "heat" that requires greater caloric burn, asks you to attempt to put the following components into your mouth every three to three-and-a-half hours:

> A Lean Protein
> A Starchy Carbohydrate
> A Fibrous Carbohydrate

Do you have to set your alarm and run to the kitchen every few hours to find the right mix of Proteins and Carbs? Of course not! You don't have to do this even anywhere close to perfectly. You just have to eat as often as possible getting the meals closer to optimal than your meals have been.

Three Important Points To Remember
• Every 3 - 3 1/2 hours, attempt to get a **Supportive Meal!**

• A **Supportive Meal** Contains A Lean Protein, Starchy Carb, and Fibrous Carb.

• **You Don't Have To Do this Perfectly!**
Just Do Better Than You're Doing Now
and You'll See Progress!

Following are some examples of supportive meal components:

Lean Proteins
Egg Whites (the yolks contain the fat and cholesterol)
Chicken Breast (dark meat chicken is much higher in fat)
Turkey Breast (ditto for turkey)
Most fresh fish and shellfish (this opens up hundreds of possibilities from lobster to tuna!)

Starchy Carbohydrates
Potatoes
Sweet Potatoes
Whole Grains
Oatmeal
Brown Rice

Fibrous Carbohydrate
Cauliflower
Broccoli
Mushrooms
Spinach
Dark Green Leafy Vegetables
Peppers
String Beans

The next question is usually, "How much?" People want measures. They want to know portions sizes, calories, grams, and other measures, none of which are simple for the average person to discern. I learned a little trick that works real well. Trust.

Trust your mind, your body, and whatever you believe the force to be that creates and maintains life. Allow your appetite to be your guide. Let me tell you about Kenny, and then I'll tell you precisely how you can trust and know "how much?"

Kenny and the "How Much" Phone calls

Kenny had been a friend of mine for several years, and while he knew what I do for a living, he never really asked me to help him get rid of the flab he'd been battling with since we met. He would sometimes ask me for tips, and of course I'd answer his questions, but he was skeptical and remained on his program which consisted of an hour a day on the stairmaster and lots of salads and baked potatoes. One day Kenny was in my office chatting with my assistant Kira while I was finishing up a phone call. He noticed some of our before and after photos on the wall. He had to ask. _"Is this for real?"_ Kira nodded. _"And this guy used to be this fat?!?"_ Kira was used to these questions. She calmly responded with a very simple, _"Yup."_ By the time I stepped out of the office, Ken was all excited. _"Just tell me what to do. I'll follow it. C'mon Phil. Why didn't you tell me? You mean these photos are for real? I'm ready. What do I do...."_

As Ken rambled on, I ushered him back into my office and set him up with a series of tapes and a program overview. Ken exited as if a bundle of fire just flared through the office and out the door! He was pumped! The next day it started. The "Kenny's on the Phone" nightmare. It started very simply. _"How much rice should I eat with my chicken?"_ Then a few minutes later, _"How much chicken?"_ There were probably 25 "Kenny's on the Phone" calls that day. The following morning he pulled into the parking lot and came up to the office with a bowl of oatmeal. _"Is this the right amount?"_

Both Kira and I assured Kenny that he has to learn to trust his body. He'd drive himself (and us) completely crazy if he kept measuring every meal. The first week, confusion is to be expected, however, within the second week your appetite will become extremely supportive. _"You'll just know."_

We made it through the week of "Kenny's on the Phone" and finally, it "kicked in." The happy ending . . . Ken transformed his body, looked fantastic on his wedding day, and became a walking, living, breathing testimonial for "the Body Transformation Program." If you ask Kenny _"how much,"_ he'll tell you about trusting your body.

Note: If you are looking for varieties in turning this combination into "real food" in the "real world," call my offices to obtain <u>EAT! Supportive Nutrition For The Body You Love</u>, a recipe book with limitless options and tips for real life supportive nutrition. ($24.95, Great Atlantic Publishing Group). For Gourmet tasting meals, I've released <u>ENJOY!</u>, featuring supportive meals worthy of any fit chef. ($19.95, Great Atlantic Publishing Group). To order call 1 800 552-1998

Simple Step #3: Limit Fat But Recognize and Avoid Sugar

You know already that you want to limit fat intake. Not "eliminate," but "limit." Keep in mind, your chicken breast has fat in it. That nice piece of salmon, while a supportive protein, contains some good fish oils. Those are fats. To simplify the process of limiting fat, I'd say just avoid those foods high in saturated fats (fats that are solid at room temperature such as the fat on a marbled steak or butter), keep away from foods that contain the word "hydrogenated" on their ingredient labels (such as margarine), and avoid adding fats unnecessarily to foods.

We have all heard that the average American needs to reduce fat intake, but still we have as a nation grown fatter. Obviously there's more to the puzzle than just knowing we should reduce fat intake.

When I first began systemizing and implementing my *Body Transformation Program*, I conducted the sessions in small groups. I'd ask the clients to stop by a supermarket and pick out a few foods they thought would help them in their quest for new bodies. Inevitably "Fat-Free" cookies, cakes, and snack foods would creep into their shopping carts.

I believe one of the greatest realizations for those frustrated by their weight loss flops was the amount of sugar they were consuming. I've seen reports that indicate the average American consumes over 150 pounds of sugar each year! Keep in mind, that's the "average" American. Imagine how much sugar someone who makes sugar a staple consumes! The shock of the massive sugar consumption taking place in this country was usually exceeded in these groups only by the shock of the impact simple sugar has on destroying the body's momentary capacity to release fat. I'll make it simple. Every time you put a simple sugar in your body, you literally "lock in" stored bodyfat.

Let's go back to the snack foods. If you have a box of your favorite fat-free cookies handy, grab the box and glance at the fine print following the word, "Ingredients." Sugar is quite likely the first ingredient listed, and if it's not first, it's pretty high up on the list. If it doesn't say the word, "sugar," that doesn't mean it's sugar free. Glucose, fructose, corn syrup, barley malt, honey, sucrose, and fruit extracts are all examples of simple sugars.

I'm sure you've heard of the hormone insulin. You probably heard it mentioned in reference to diabetes. Diabetes is a blood sugar irregularity and insulin is the hormone that regulates sugar transport and storage. It is vital for normal energy production. In healthy individuals, insulin is produced by the pancreas in amounts dictated by blood sugar levels.

When you eat a complex carbohydrate, such as a potato, you have really taken in long chains of sugar linked together. The "chains" of sugar, as opposed to the simple sugars in candy and cookies, are the reason those more supportive carbohydrates are termed "complex." As the carbohydrates pass through your digestive tract, the chains are slowly broken apart sending a slow release of sugar into the bloodstream. When, in contrast to the complex carbs, you ingest simple sugars, all of those sugars are absorbed at once, thus, for the moment you have high blood sugar. The pancreas is signaled to produce more insulin and that insulin than transports the excess sugar out of the bloodstream and into the muscles and liver to be stored.

There is another hormone you might not have heard of. Glucagon. While insulin is a "storage" hormone, glucagon is an energy releasing hormone. Glucagon's job is to free up bodyfat if you are going to burn it as fuel. The catch here is, the pancreas does a bit of a balancing act, and when it is called upon to produce more insulin due to an elevation in blood sugar, it backs off its production of glucagon. No glucagon, no fat release! No fat release, no fat burning! You're starting to see the obstacle sugar ingestion presents, aren't you? Good. Let me keep going.

When you experience that sugar induced blood sugar elevation, your pancreas sort of overreacts and sends out more insulin than required. While your blood sugar is up in the stratosphere, you may feel a sense of what you perceive to be energy. That sugar rush is short term, for as soon as the new insulin begins getting that blood sugar down, it overcompensates and leaves you with residual low blood sugar. You may feel weak and tired. Here's the crazy part. In an effort now to restore your blood sugar to normal, your body sends out signals which are interpreted in your brain as *"Go Eat Sugar!"* Thus, when you eat sugar, you crave sugar!

If you are a bit of a sugarholic, I know you might find this hard to believe, but I'll stake my reputation on it. Give up simple sugar for three days, eat the way I'm recommending, exercise as I'm going to recommend, and your sugar cravings can be written off as a memory. I'm not going to tell you that you'll never want for cheesecake again, and I'd never tell you to give up any food you like completely, but you will find your tastes and appetite become far more supportive if you minimize what might be a very high intake of that sabotaging simple sugar!

OK, so cookies aren't the best. Ice cream is not going to pass the sugar test. Pastries seem to have dropped down to the bottom of the "supportive" list. How about pretzels? Low-fat eaters have known pretzels are a great snack food, right? Well, let's take a look at . . . you should know by now . . . the ingredients. Sugar? Probably not, but you'll probably find Ingredient #1 to be "Enriched," "Bleached" or "Processed" flour. Flour usually begins as a very nutritious whole grain. The words I just listed really mean that a big old machine did lot of the "work" (remember, the calorie burning heat production in the act of digesting?) your body could benefit from. Many of the beneficial nutrients are lost in processing. Since those calories are still "in" calories, meaning you're still going to consume four calories per gram (carbohydrates), they do count, yet you lose out on that 10% metabolic boost more supportive complex carbs would provide. These "processed" or "refined" carbohydrates are easily converted into triglycerides, thus, it is not unlikely that those "healthy" pretzels wind up as stored fat on your hips or your waistline. Does that mean pretzels are bad? No, not if you enjoy them. Don't, however, believe that they're going to assist you in your quest for leanness.

Those refined carbs, or "empty calories," are also the ingredients of most supermarket bought breads and baked foods. We'll get further into reading and understanding food labels in the next section.

Wayne, The Sugar Eater!

In one of my early Body Transformation Program group sessions, I had the opportunity to meet Wayne Gregory. Wayne had been overweight for most of his life. He had been anything but lazy. In fact, Wayne tried diet after diet and when I met him, he was involved in an exercise program which had him performing aerobic exercise between 45 and 90 minutes every single day! Wayne decided he was just stuck in a fat body. He came to me as a last hope. I remember when I was discussing exercise, Wayne was nodding his head and taking notes. He was very accepting of everything I went over, until . . . I brought up the topic of sugar! Wayne looked up as if he had been stung. I had to ask. _"What's wrong?"_ Wayne responded, _"I eat healthy. It's just that, well . . . I "need" sugar. If I don't have my snack before bed, I can't sleep!"_ Sure enough, Wayne was buying the fat-free cookies and ice creams and including them as integral crutches in sticking to his low-calorie diets. _"Wayne, I'm going to ask you to trust me. Eat the way I'm suggesting and exercise as I'm outlining in the program. Avoid sugar for three days. The first day you might get a slight headache and feel fatigued. The second day the headache may worsen and you might experience insomnia, and the third day might be the worst day of all. Then, you'll be craving free! Your energy will stabilize, and you'll begin releasing fat at a rate you'll_ *find shocking!"* Four days later Wayne called. He started, *"Phil, I'm getting cravings."* I was upset. I began to attack. *"Well, then you didn't do what I said. You're still eating sugar...."* *"Phil, hold on,"* Wayne interrupted. *"I know this sounds crazy, but, I'm craving brown rice!"* Several weeks later an amazingly reduced Wayne walked into my office and handed me a belt. That was the first. A few weeks after that he brought in another belt as his waist was continuing to shrink. Several weeks after that Wayne began a new life as a physically fit man, a life which had him in better shape at age 48 than he was in the military almost 30 years earlier! He continues to express his gratitude . . . and it all started with knocking out that saboteur of fat loss . . . SUGAR!

Simple Step #4: Don't Be Fooled by Labels and Hype – Buy and Eat Supportive Food!

Food manufacturers know you. They make it a point to. The words that they put on their labels are words that are intended to compel you to make a purchase. Thus, you'll find the words, Light, Low-Fat, Fat-Free, Lean, and Healthy all over foods that might not have the slightest resemblance to the foods I've outlined as Supportive.

The first suggestion I'll make is to find a natural market or health food store and purchase your produce, meats, poultry, and fish there. If such a store is not accessible or convenient, I'll suggest limiting most of your purchases to the perimeter of the traditional supermarket. With that as the first suggestion, you'll then help your results dramatically once you learn to see through what I believe to be food label fraud.

%DV
On food labels you'll find nutrient listings supposedly reporting fat, carbohydrate, and protein content. On each line you'll find a percentage. At the top of the percentage column it reads % DV with a little asterisk. If you look at the footnote that asterisk leads you to it tells you that you're looking at the % Daily Value. What in the world is that? It's a meaningless number that tricks many people into believing that high fat foods are lower in fat than they really are, that's what it is!

If you shift your eyes down to the very fine print that the asterisk sort of directs you to, you'll find it says, "Percent Daily Values are based on a 2000 calorie diet." First of all, who says a 2,000 calorie diet has anything to do with your metabolism or your lifestyle? Secondly, even if you were following a 2,000 calorie diet, are you supposed to keep a running total adding up percentages in all the foods you eat? It's absurd! % DV does two things. Firstly, it allows food manufacturers to put a % value next to fat content. Since for many years Americans were told to limit fat intake to 30% of their diet (a percentage I believe far too high), consumers will simply glance at the "fat" line and if they see a percentage below 30, believe a food to be a wise choice. That's why "Reduced Fat" Peanut butter can have about half of its calories from fat and still sport a 19% reading on the "fat" line. It's 19% DV. It's 19% nonsense. It's a high fat food!!!!!

The best way to handle % DV . . . ignore it completely!

Fat-Free

Many food labels have the words "fat-free" blaring out on the front for one reason and one reason only. Those words sell products. Does it have anything to do with the contents? In far too many cases, I'd have to say absolutely not! Walk into the grocery store, or perhaps only as far as your fridge, and pick up one of those "Fat-Free" butter substitutes. Look at the ingredients. You'll likely find the only ingredient of substance to be a hydrogenated oil. Hydrogenated oils are pure fat! So, how do they get away with calling pure fat "fat-free?" The labeling laws seem to be created with massive holes which allow the food labelers to (shall I be polite?) . . . . mislead. (If I were to be more "to the point" I'd say "lie.") The loophole usually involves the serving size. If there is less than 1/2 gram of fat in a serving (note the words, "in a serving"), a food can be labeled "fat-free." The law, however, does not define a serving size. By making the serving size, in its entirety, less than 1/2 gram, any food can be labeled "Fat-Free!" Yes, even a pure fat!

90% Fat-Free?

If you were to eat a stick of butter (please don't do it!) you'd be taking in 100% of your calories from fat. If you mixed the butter in water and drank the solution, since water doesn't have any calories, you'd still be getting all of your calories from fat. If, however, we were going to market the butter - water solution, and we wanted to reach consumers who were concerned about their weight, we wouldn't sell a whole lot if we put the words, "100% of calories from FAT" on the label. We could therefore be just a bit tricky. We could modify the amount of water to make the "solution" as "fat-free" as we'd like. For example, if we put equal amounts of butter and water, we could label the solution, "50% Fat-Free." Sure, 100% of the calories would be from fat, but we'd be within the realm of the law. Hmm. 50% doesn't sound that good. How about if we add more water until we create a solution with all of its calories from fat that we can label 90% Fat-Free? Good idea? Maybe if you are in the business of selling high fat - water solutions it would be. If you were on the other end of it, a consumer believing 90% fat free indicates a low-fat choice, you would likely be deceived.

Guess what. The turkey in the grocery store labeled lean? Most of what's in that container is water. That's why they can label a meat which obtains near half of its calories from fat as "93% fat free!" (Note: be certain the "lean" turkey you choose is actually turkey breast meat). 2% fat milk is often looked at by unknowing consumers as a low-fat choice. Examine the label and do the math. You'll find that near 40% of the calories are fat calories! Now you understand. Milk is primarily water by volume, thus, it leaves an open door for widespread deception.

So How Do You See Through This Deception?
On any food label they are required to list ingredients in descending order of abundance. Skip the big print and go right to the ingredients. If any item on that ingredient list has fat in it (oil, lard, butter, whole milk, etc.), you can not be looking at a fat-free food regardless of what the big print promises.

They are also required to list the number of calories per serving and the number of calories from fat. First examine the serving size to make certain it is more than 1/2 gram. Then, ignore % DV and any advertising words on the front of the label. Divide the number of fat calories by the number of calories to determine what percentage of the food is fat. For example, if a label indicates 120 calories per serving, 30 calories from fat, 30 divided by 120 = .25 indicating that the food would obtain 25% of its calories from fat.

I'd suggest trying to keep overall fat intake down to 15% of your caloric intake and avoiding any foods that get more than 25% of their calories from fat.

Sugar Free?
By now you're becoming far less trusting of labels. Good! You're protected. We also know the impact simple sugars have on your fat loss capacity. Look at labels and avoid the foods with substantial amounts of sugar. Simple sugars can have many names. I've seen labels indicate that the enclosed cookies were "sugar Free" yet the most prominent ingredient was fructose. Sure, it's fruit sugar, and yes they can call it natural, but . . . . a rose by any other name is still a rose. A simple sugar by any other name . . . you get the point. Allow me to repeat a sentence from the earlier chapter where I discussed snack foods. Glucose, fructose, corn syrup, barley malt, honey, sucrose, and fruit extracts are all examples of simple sugars.

Can You Ever Eat Those Fats and Sugars You Love?
Hey, it's the real world! I love a good pizza as much as anyone. I also have a true passion for ice cream. I've learned that if you tell anyone what they can't eat, they begin to think about whatever it is that you're asking them to avoid! Sooner or later, they give in and feel guilty! That's why I encourage people to choose one day per week, and on that day, give in! Since you're spending six days speeding metabolism, "the Cheat Day" is well justified, and since the body's getting better at burning through food, your putting the less supportive stuff into a much "hotter" furnace. Enjoy your cheat days! Interestingly enough, when you start to eat supportively, you'll find your tastes change. You'll find you feel more energetic. You'll find that even with permission, you begin to have less interest in cheat days! You'll find with control of your metabolism, life just gets better and better!

Simple Step #5: Exercise Aerobically, but in Moderation

You might have been led to believe that "aerobic exercise" burns fat. That might be true, but then again, it might not! Confused!?!? I don't blame you. Don't worry. I'll clear it up right here and now.

Perhaps in the past you've tried to reduce, tone up, or lose weight by employing the use of a treadmill, stairclimber, or exercise bike. Maybe you tried walking, jogging, or aerobic dancing. You lost weight, you eventually backed off on the exercise, and the weight came back. Even while you lost the weight, it's quite possible you didn't develop the lean toned look you'd hoped for. Why? Because you might have been feeding off of muscle!

Let me first explain the definition of aerobic. In a textbook sense, it means, "with oxygen." Does that mean there are some types of exercise in which we don't use oxygen? Of course not. We'd be dead! Let me clarify the definition for you.

"Aerobic," for our purposes, more accurately indicates that we can "meet the demand" for oxygen. If I were to ask you to run as fast as you can, and then I were to run right along side you and keep yelling in your ear, *"Faster! I want you to run faster!"* it wouldn't take long before you pooped out and collapsed (or you lost your hearing in one ear!). You would reach the "anaerobic threshold," the point at which your heart could no longer supply enough oxygen to meet the muscles' demand. Anything, therefore, that you can continue for five, ten, twenty minutes, or more, would be aerobic. If you are reading this seated in a chair, you are in an "aerobic state!" You are meeting the demand for oxygen!

Anytime you are in an aerobic state, your body has two options for fuel. It can burn fat, and / or, it can burn sugar! If you have not made fat an available fuel source, your body will have only one option during aerobic exercise. Sugar. If your blood sugar is fluctuating due to going long periods of time without consuming supportive meals, fat release will be compromised. If you consume simple sugars, fat release will be compromised. If you don't take in enough calories to support your activity, your body will actually "cling" to fat. Any of those conditions will cause any aerobic movement to seek out sugar as a fuel source. You can see that aerobic exercise may not tap into your stored fat at all!

Where does it get the sugar to burn? Well, the complex carbs that you consume are slowly converted into glucose and stored in the muscles as "glycogen." Glycogen, in essence, is "stored sugar" in muscles as a fuel reserve. Your glycogen supply is limited and if you don't eat sufficiently to keep those stores full, your aerobic session may exhaust your "stored sugar." If you exhaust your supply of glycogen your body will tap into muscle stores to create its own fuel. It actually converts some amino acids into sugars. The only way it can get at those amino acids is to break apart muscle tissue. Thus, it becomes possible to "exercise away muscle tissue!" You by now understand that will have a long term negative effect making your body more efficient at storing fat!

You absolutely want to include aerobic exercise in your Body Transformation Program. It's just that you want to make certain you don't feed off of that valuable lean body mass. Remember, if you get the other pieces of the puzzle right, you can feed off of fat anytime you're in an aerobic state. That includes right now! I suggest starting out with only 12 minutes a day of moderate intensity aerobic exercise. That's it! You can always progress!

Simple Step #6: Challenge and Protect Muscle!

Muscle. I've mentioned it quite a few times. There are many misconceptions associated with the word and the emergence of drug enhanced over-sized muscle obsessed bodybuilders has furthered many of those misconceptions among the general public. The fact is, we all should place the utmost value on muscle!

Muscle is metabolism! It's the only part of your body that burns calories!

Q: Wait a minute Phil, what about the heart? Doesn't that burn calories?

A: Of course it does! Guess what the heart is. You guessed it. A muscle!

Muscle produces heat. Muscle protects the internal organs and provides movement. Lose a bit of muscle and health and metabolism begin a decline.

The good news is, it's simple to "protect muscle." You already know that you don't want to starve away or exercise away muscle. Now you want to build some, even a bit, because that increases the size of the fat burning furnace. In order to protect that vital furnace, ask your muscles to resist. That's it! Simply ask them to do a bit more than they're used to and then allow them to rest. That doesn't mean you need spend hours upon hours sweating in a gym. It means exactly what it sounds like. Challenge your muscles several times per week and, as long as your nutrition is supportive, you're protected!

There are so many options for providing this muscle challenge I could not even attempt to list them here. I would create an entire encyclopedia in the process. In my TRANSFORM! book, I do list and explain enough options for anyone to design their own supportive routine. For now, if you are not accustomed to resistance exercise, I'd suggest investing less than $20 in a couple of light pairs of dumbbells and finding a fitness professional who can design a very simple 15-minute routine which can be performed 3 times per week in your own home. You can call my office for other options if you'd like. I've made available limitless options for those who are free to travel to my fitness locations as well as those who are anywhere else in the world (that about covers everyone, doesn't it?).

If you are already exercising with resistance, modifications in the six other steps will make your present exercise far more productive and the payoff will thrill you!

Simple Step #7: Change the Focus of Your Exercise Regularly for Ongoing Progress

The body is amazingly adaptive. In fact, when it sheds fat due to a change in eating and activity, it is actually adapting to a new stimulus. If, therefore, you continue the same exact workouts every day of every week of every month, you'll hit what exercisers refer to as, The Plateau. If your body were going to speak to you in a language you readily understand, the Plateau would be translated as, *"I can handle this. I don't need to change anymore."*

In order to prevent *the Plateau* from creeping up on you, it's important to modify the way that you stimulate your muscles. There are several ways of varying the focus. I've used the concept of "Cycle Training" as the cornerstone of my Body Transformation Programs. Rather than staying with the same regimen, you "cycle" the exercise regimen employing a different focus during different periods within the cycle. Here are two examples.

Example #1:
Two Weeks of Strength Training focusing on Muscle Growth
Six Weeks of Muscle Shaping employing more repetitions with lighter weights
Four Weeks of Endurance Training With Shortened Rest Periods
One Week of Recuperative Activity

Example #1 offers a 13-week cycle which can be repeated four times a year.

Example #2
One Week of Metabolism Boosting Focus
One Week of Muscle Endurance and Fat Release
One Week of Intense Fat Burning

That would provide a 3-week cycle which can be repeated on an ongoing basis until leanness and weight loss goals are achieved

Note in both of those examples the focus is changed systematically to avoid *the Plateau*. Again, herein I want you to understand the concept. If you're no longer making progress with a routine that used to work, you should now understand why. If you want specific details on designing a Cycle Training routine, I'll again refer you to my TRANSFORM! book or program and/or a meeting with a qualified fitness professional.

The "Answer" to the most common Questions:

Q: Am I too Old?

A: This is a simple one. No. If you are still processing food, if you are still able to move, than you can apply the principles that will allow you to improve. How much you can improve is going to be a very individual issue, however, I assure you that you can be in better shape next month than you are right now, and that improvement can absolutely continue from that point forward! In fact, Donna Michaels, a good friend of mine and a fitness professional who has achieved the best shape of her life after the age of 50, is continuing to find better health and fitness with each decade. She believes that aging as we know it, may be a myth or a mistake, and I'm inclined to agree!

Q: Am I too Fat?

A: I've already received scores of letters and thank you's from individuals who have lost well over 100 pounds each! They all reported dramatic improvements to nearly every aspect of their lives. Each one of those people, at some time, believed he or she was "too fat" for this to work. The fact is, what a professional athlete does, in concept, to put the body in a state where it is willing to burn fat, is exactly the same (in concept) as any human must do to shed fat. The more fat you have, the greater the period of time required to achieve a lean body, but focusing on simply being in better shape today than last month can take anyone to the point of a lean, toned, healthy body given the luxury of the true technology (the Seven Steps) and time.

Q: Does liposuction work?

A: Sure. It works to remove subcutaneous fat deposits, however, it doesn't do anything to change the machine. A metabolism that accumulated fat in the first place will likely redeposit fat stores if fat is removed surgically. On the other hand, if you apply the Seven Steps, you not only rid the body of fat, but you completely alter the mechanism that stored fat in the first place minimizing the odds of it ever coming back. Liposuction, as all cosmetic surgery, is a surgical procedure and with any such procedure come risks. Liposuction should not be viewed as a solution to a body that is carrying too high a level of bodyfat.

Q: What About Supplements?

A: There are some supplements that have value, however, supplements are often mis-marketed as "solutions." In order for a supplement to have value, it's essential that "the foundation" is firmly laid in place, and that foundation lies in learning to balance the right nutrition with a result oriented exercise program.

Q: *What About the New Hormonal Products?*

A law was passed recently that allows "anything found naturally in the human body or in plants" to be sold as a supplement rather than classified as a drug. That brought an explosion of "hormonal" products ranging from melatonin as a sleep inducer to DHEA as a rejuvenator and a ticket to recapturing youth. While some of these products may be relatively safe in small dosages, and they may have short term value, playing around with the body's endocrine or hormonal production often has a rebound effect in which natural hormonal production is altered. I would urge you to avoid these products or to check with a doctor very well versed in the endocrine system before randomly attempting supplementation with any hormonal products.

Q: *Is Creatine going to add muscle?*

A: Creatine Monohydrate is one of the few supplements I have endorsed as having true value if muscle size and strength are goals. Many new products make outrageous claims leading you to believe there is some magic in creatine. Ingesting creatine monohydrate will likely have two effects in the well-nourished exerciser. Firstly, it will attract more water into each muscle cell increasing overall muscle volume. Secondly, it will likely lead to greater storage of creatine phosphate, a muscle fuel source, leading to enhanced training performance. I've seen the most consistent results by beginning with 20 grams of Creatine Monohydrate per day broken into four 5-gram servings. It's a powder and can be mixed in water or dilute fruit juice. After the first 5 days, 5 grams per day appears to be sufficient. One heaping teaspoon approximates 5 grams. As a footnote, you don't "need" creatine, it is only a supplement, and when you stop using it, expect to lose some of the effect.

Q: *Should I use Protein Supplements?*

Protein is the nutrient that leads to the maintenance and building of every cell in your body. That doesn't mean that eating more protein leads to more cells as many protein sellers would lead you to believe. You should, as you by now know, attempt to get supportive meals. In the event that supportive meals are not convenient, supplement powders that contain protein, complex carbs, a small amount of essential fats, and a complete profile of vitamins and minerals would be the next best thing. If you do use a protein only supplement, it should be consumed with food that constitutes the other nutrients such as a protein drink with a salad or a protein drink with a potato and some fibrous vegetables. In today's world, with all of us trying to juggle busy schedules, I do find that maintaining a supportive nutrition program usually requires the use of some supplemental meals. For that reason I created the EAT! Formula Metabolism Enhancer. It offer supportive nutrition in a powder (mix with water) when a meal is not convenient.

Q: What if I'm a vegetarian?

A: The greatest challenge I find for vegetarians attempting to follow a Supportive Nutrition Program is in obtaining enough complete proteins to maintain muscle. While many vegetable foods do contain protein, most are lacking in the amounts of some vital amino acids needed for growth, thus cell maintenance and growth becomes a challenge. There are specific combinations of non-animal foods that complement each other to provide more valuable proteins such as consuming black beans with brown rice. It is therefore important for a "vegan," or a strict vegetarian to become a bit more educated in nutrition than someone willing to include some animal products. The use of a soy protein supplement can help as soy is the closest to animal products in its protein value. If you are a lacto-ovo vegetarian, the use of non-fat dairy products can supply your proteins. If you are willing to eat fish, the options are limitless. Anybody can take control of metabolism and reshape their body any way they want to. If you are vegetarian for moral and ethical reasons, I would not attempt to modify your commitment. If, on the other hand, you had "health" in mind, and a little at a time you eliminated foods without finding sufficient nutrient replacement, you might want to re-examine your choices. Perhaps making a few allowances will allow you to build better cells, stronger bones, and a healthier metabolism fueling much enhanced immune, circulatory, and respiratory function.

Q: What About Fruit? Healthy?

A: This is one of the most common questions I receive and my answer is often take out of context. I'll make it very simple. Fruits are very healthy. They're very water dense, high in vitamins and minerals, and chock full of great taste. They are also high in simple sugar. That makes them less than ideal if you're looking to release as much fat as possible. With all that you now know about sugar, you might see some value in cutting back a bit if your diet is very high in high sugar fruits.

Q: How Do I Get Started?

A: Review the Seven Steps. If this is all new to you, I'd spend one week just examining the labels of the foods you eat and beginning to identify which foods are lean proteins, which are starchy carbs and which are fibrous carbs. Also identify and work on weaning away from simple sugars. In that first week commit to 12 minutes per day of walking or some type of moderate aerobic exercise. In the second week try to make certain each meal has a lean protein, starchy carb, and fibrous carb. Rather than seeking out perfection, just try to do "better than you've done in the past." When that becomes comfortable, attempt to get "Supportive Meals" every 3 - 3 1/2 hours, again seeking nothing more than progress. The final step is to implement a resistance training program and with that in place you are applying the technology that will allow you to shed fat and develop a lean, toned, body.

Q: What should I do for resistance training?

Actually, it can be as simple as doing squats or lunges, pushups, and some type of chinning or pullup movement without any weight at all. My suggestion is to use dumbbells and find a resource that will teach you a few basic movements which when combined work all of the major muscles in the body. Make certain you "vary" the focus of your training, preferably with a plan. You might train for two weeks using heavier weights and then two weeks using lighter weights for greater numbers of repetitions. This book is not intended to be a strength training guide. My TRANSFORM! Program teaches people how to design a resistance training program that will last them a lifetime. There are other resources available. If you have never done resistance training, a single session with a qualified fitness professional might be a good idea.

Q: What is the 17-Day Program?

In advance copies of the Answer, I included information about my 17-Day Program. I started conducting it in small groups where people would attend four group sessions over a three-week period. More than anything else, it is 17 days of application of the Seven Simple Steps and serves as an educational process. It is not "magic," but as all of my programs, it empowers people to take control of their lives and metabolisms. I marketed it toward that audience that believes that 17 weeks, the time it takes to go through my Body Transformation Program is an eternity. The fact is, the 17-Week program is far more comprehensive and all-inclusive. The 17-Days allows the foundation to become ingrained as you watch your body make some positive changes.

Q: How do I decide between the 17-Day Program and the full Body Transformation Program?

If you're ready to make an all out commitment, and you fully understand the virtues of supportive nutrition, moderate aerobic exercise, and a concern for muscle, the complete Body Transformation is all you'll ever need to shape your body any way you want to. If you want to "test the waters," if you think 17 weeks sounds like forever, and if you're not at the point that you want to focus your attention on 3 hours of video and a commitment to making some very powerful changes, the 17-Day Program will be the kick start you need!

Who is Phil Kaplan . . . and Why Should We Believe Him?

Early on in the text I promised you I'd touch on my story. I'll keep it brief. Belief, however, is a vital prerequisite to changing your body and with all of the so-called options being flung around labeled as solutions, apprehension is only natural. If you question anybody selling you a fitness or weight loss solution, I applaud you! In fact, I've devoted my life to getting people to raise that, "Why Should I Believe You," question. If enough people begin to question, it's only a matter of time until "The Answer" reaches everyone.

In attempts to keep it brief, I'll simply mention that I started in this industry as a fitness instructor with a paycheck amounting to $4.25 per hour at Jack La Lanne Health Spas in Little Neck, New York. After experiencing very positive changes in my own life due to accepting an exercise lifestyle, I was truly passionate about sharing it with others. Over a period of years, I worked my way through the health club ranks to become a National Director for the largest health club chain in the country and expand my physiology education to the point that 17 certifications hung on my wall. American Council on Exercise. National Strength & Conditioning Association, etc. My frustration grew daily. While I was helping a tiny segment of the membership find results, and following the conventional course of accumulating and documenting knowledge, the huge corporation was simply selling memberships and most people who were enrolling would fail to achieve any result at all!

I finally decided to begin my own Personal Training company. Having moved to South Florida, I found clients ranging from celebrities in town for appearances to plain ordinary people who wanted to make a change. It took me a while to catch on, but I soon realized the only reason people were failing . . . they were being misled! Worst of all, they didn't know they were being misled so they were blaming themselves!

I went back to working with health clubs, this time as a consultant, teaching club owners to prosper by delivering results and meeting the needs of others. I established a position within the industry as the consultant who delivers and "Influences With Integrity." I was reaching more people, but in the grand scheme of things, I still felt that I wasn't making a dent. Diets were ripping people off to the tune of billions of dollars per year and I was only reaching a select few. I began to explore outside of conventional education. If anyone anywhere was achieving true results, I wanted to learn what they were doing.

I studied with and learned from world renowned scientists, biochemists, bodybuilders, trainers, coaches, etc. and soon found a strong link among all of them. They were educating people in the essential combination of the right nutrition, aerobic exercise, and a concern for muscle. As I explored further, I began to uncover fraud and deception in ads, programs, and even in some of the most financially successful weight loss offerings. I had to spread the truth! It became more than a passion, it became a driving mission.

I wrote a book, Mind & Muscle: Fitness For All of You. The publishers didn't want it. They wanted me to say, "it's quick, it's easy, it works like magic!" Instead I did something unique. I told the truth and that wasn't appealing to book publishers at the time. They wanted hype. Some small publishers made me offers, but I knew I had to go outside of conventional channels. After all, too many dollars would be at risk if the truth found its way to the general public! Diets? Fat-Free foods? Miracle supplements? We're talking about a whole lot of money which book publishers were hesitant to go up against.

I started speaking anywhere I could find people who were willing to listen. Bookstores. Schools. Conventions. As I spoke with greater conviction and frequency, more and more people started to listen. Through a complex and fateful chain of events, I was invited to begin broadcasting a radio show, The Mind & Muscle Fitness Hour.

More and more people were listening, and I soon had a regular audience. They were applying the information I was sharing, and they were transform-ing! I started telling listeners about my book, and soon, without knowing anything about radio broadcasting or book promoting, I sold 5,000 Mind & Muscle books! That's when calls and letters starting pouring in with great stories of physical change. The "thanks, Phil, you changed my body" letters piled up high and I finally felt I was making a difference. I started conducting seminars and group programs and began gaining quite a reputation with the 100% success rate my Body Transformation Program maintained. It wasn't long before I was invited to appear as a guest on TV shows ranging from local and regional news to Good Day New York, AM Buffalo, and Hard Copy. The phone was ringing off the hook. People wanted me for seminars, radio appearances, and TV shows nationwide. I was finally making a difference. That's when it all went haywire! Totally flat-out off-the-wall haywire!

The infomercial companies began soliciting me. "C'mon, Phil. You'll make a few million dollars." They didn't seem to care what the product was, they just knew I was reaching people and making phones ring.

I told you I'd make the long story short. The story that unfolded from this point forward is shocking. It's filled with intrigue, with legal battles, millions of dollars, deception, mega-corporations, massive television shoots, and maybe even the slightest bit of sex and violence (hey, I said maybe. I'm just warming you up for when they make the full length movie!). I know that this is not the forum for the story, so I'll refine the whole escapade into a single sterile paragraph.

I signed a contract with a company that soon owned my name, my image, and my program. They wanted me to "hype" and "pitch" and make the program sound magical and I insisted on telling the truth. The battle that ensued nearly drained me emotionally, financially, and physically. I kept going. Another infomercial company helped me get out of my messy deal, and sure enough . . . it was out of the frying pan and into the fire. The people who were simply applying what I was teaching them, those who kept thanking me, gave me the strength to keep going. The thank you's, the knowledge that it was "working," helped me believe I was doing the right thing as the media powers drained me and fought tooth and nail to get me to sacrifice my commitment to truth and integrity. I believe "the right thing" has its payoff, and in that I keep driving forward, breaking down walls and spreading the word (end of single, sterile paragraph that condensed "the whole story).

Dr. Anthony Abbott is not well known outside of fitness circles, however, he is far and away one of the most respected individuals within the fitness educational circles. He honored me at a banquet for my battle against fitness misinformation and came up with a line that struck me. "Phil doesn't tell people what they want to hear, he tells them what they need to hear." The marketers of products, programs, infomercials, etc., have learned to cash in by telling people what they want to hear. Food labelers and supplement sellers have cashed in by altering perception and make people believe falsehoods. Many of the large health club chains have sent out the message, "Join and you'll be fit" full knowing most of their members never even show up!

It became a true battle, but through my appearances and articles, I'm reaching people at a steady rate. I wrote *the Answer* to introduce those of you who haven't yet gone through my Program to find and accept the true technology of physical change. I'm proud and thankful that I've now reached you!

To contact Phil Kaplan's South Florida offices

Phil Kaplan's Fitness, 1304 SW 160th Ave, #337, Ft Lauderdale, FL 33326
Telephone (954) 389-0280   Fax (954) 742-3173
Website: http://philkaplan.com   E-mail: phil@philkaplan.com

Available Through Phil's offices:

• **TRANSFORM!** The book. 368 pages. $39.95

• **EAT! Supportive Nutrition For The Body You Love!** Recipes and detailed tips for making Supportive Nutrition simple. $24.95

• **Mind & Muscle: Fitness For All of You.** 1994 182 pgs. $24.95

• **Body Transformation Seminar Video.** 2 tapes. 3 hrs. $39.95

• **The Complete Body Transformation Program.** The program that has brought Phil worldwide acclaim. It's all in here! TRANSFORM!, the EAT! recipe book, the Body Transformation seminar video, six audio cassettes, and the complete 17-Week Body Transformation Program with a Journal and Exercise Log. $189.95

• **Resolutions CD.** Phil speaks to you and "makes sense." $19.95

• **ENJOY!** Supportive Gourmet Recipes. $19.95

• **EAT! Metabolism Enhancer.** Vanilla or Chocolate. 1 lb. $24.95 Protein, carbs, vitamins, minerals, in a delicious powder for a supportive shake when a meal is not convenient.

• **The Fitness Professional's "Profit 2000" package** featuring Phil's booklet on "influence" in today's confusing fitness market place and 2 hours of audio cassette material teaching fitness professionals to prosper by sharing the true technology of physical change. Learn how to help others get results! $129.00

To Order Products call Phil's order line TOLL-FREE:
1 800-552-1998

For Personal Consultations or Seminars contact
Phil Kaplan and his staff at (954) 389-0280

In This Special Edition of The Answer . . .

The 17-Day Program is Included!

17 Days!

SPECIAL BONUS:

The "Answer" 17- Day Fitness Solution!

In the pages that follow you'll find the outline and overview of the newest Program by Phil Kaplan.

Get Fit in only 17 Days!

Read that headline. Catchy, isn't it? In fact, it's just the type of headline that would have raised my blood pressure a few notches. Until now that is! Can you get fit in 17 days? Hmmm. It depends how you look at it.

For years my blood would boil whenever I'd see those "Lose 30 pounds in 30 days" flyers pasted up all over walls and telephone poles. I knew as more and more people were exposed to those flyers, more and more people would waste money on ineffective solutions. That offered a massive challenge for me. If I put a flyer right next to each and every one of those "30-day" pages, mine would have to say, "Get Fit in 17 Weeks." My Body Transformation Program provides the true technology of physical change and walks people through a 17-week transformation. Now think about it. If you looked at the flyers, side by side, and asked the question, "30 days or 17 weeks?" would anybody choose 17 weeks? Of course not! For those who were seeking "The Answer," and believed quick and permanent weight loss could be one and the same, the shorter the time, the greater the appeal. The unfortunate reality is that nobody will find the lifetime results they seek in 30 days.

I thought hard, and thought harder, and my brain was burning more and more calories when I came up with the concept of the 17-day program. Could I help someone to lose weight in 17 days? Of course! Could I make that weight loss permanent by ensuring it's "fat loss?" Absolutely! Could I guarantee a number of pounds, rival that number with "30," and beat the "30-dayers" at their own game? Nope. It's just not possible. If I was going to remain honest, ethical, and maintain my stand-alone success rate, I wasn't about to cross the borders of ethics and morality. I could, however, within a 17-day period, educate people, empower them, and teach them about the Synergy thousands have used in my 17-week program. I could make sure they saw evidence of progress in the way their bodies looked . . . and . . . yes . . . on the scale as well. Evidence of progress might not equate to "30 pounds," but it would erase their flawed beliefs and teach them how to keep that evidence going until they finally loved their new bodies. I got to work.

Following you'll find the result. 17 days of physical change. You will lose fat. You will boost metabolism. You will increase tone. You must simply understand that it's a gradual process, and the first 17 days will be followed by the next. Master, however, this 17 Day technology and you will have the power to completely redesign your physical destiny!

I won't go into long explanations. In remaining with my goals in writing "The Answer," I want to keep this brief enough for you to read in a single sitting.

I'll simply outline the nutrition and exercise guidelines that will provide the power for you to experience 17 days of positive physical change!

I have also recorded a CD called "Resolutions." It is designed to act as a strong complement to this program. If you don't yet have it . . . I'll make a suggestion. Get it! Once you understand everything outlined herein, you can simply apply the 17-day program, or jump right into my TRANSFORM! program, the 17-week program that brings you every aspect of the fitness and weight loss solution you've ever needed. With only the information in your hand, there isn't any excuse. Make tomorrow Day 1 . . . or if you're reading this in the morning . . . start right NOW! Prepare to TRANSFORM!

Some Definitions That Will Help You With the 17-Day Fitness Solution Program

Set - a number of repetitions of a specific movement performed in succession without rest. In other words, one set of 20 repetitions would ask you to repeat a movement with a weight twenty times before putting the weight down.

Target Heart Zone (THZ) - the heart rate range that ensures adequate intensity for cardiorespiratory improvement. It is estimated using an Age Related Formula. Subtracting your age from 220 will estimate your Maximal Heart Rate (the fastest your heart has the capacity to beat). Your THZ would be between 65% and 80% of that number (different organizations might have slightly different percentages).

$$THZ = 220 - Age \ X \ (65\% - 80\%)$$

Protein Day - a nutritional tactic that can be used to enhance fat release, however, do not do more than suggested. While a few specially placed protein days can enhance fat release, extended cutback of carbohydrates can result in metabolic slowdown. On a Protein Day, do not consume starchy carbs. In each meal, every 3 hours, have a lean protein and a small amount of vegetable (fibrous carb). Do not consume more than 100 carb calories on a protein day. Increase protein portions by 25% as compared to a standard "Supportive Nutrition" day. If ever, in the midst of a Protein Day, you feel uncomfortable, light-headed, or out of sorts, just go back to eating supportively.

Superset - two exercises are combined without rest in between. This serves to push a muscle or muscle group past it's usual point of momentary failure allowing for greater muscle stimulation and increased intensity.

Isolation Movement - a resistance exercise which focuses in on a specific muscle or muscle group. You'll find movement takes place from only one joint.

Compound Movement - a resistance exercise which brings assisting muscle groups into play to aid the primary targeted muscle. Most compound movements will require movement from more than one joint.

Momentary Muscle Failure (MMF) - the point at which a muscle can no longer complete a repetition in strict form without stopping to rest.

Days #1 - #3

In this first three days you'll already apply steps #1 - #5 of the Seven Simple Steps revealed in The Answer. Since you are getting to "know" your metabolism, and to give it a kick start, don't focus on your weight, but rather on your ability to process food.

In this first week learn to identify the true ingredients in foods and attempt to get a supportive meal every 3 - 3 1/2 hours. If at first it's challenging, opt for three supportive meals and two meal replacement shakes each day. (Look for a meal replacement that uses either egg protein, milk protein isolates, or whey and is free from saturated or hydrogenated fats and contains very little or absolutely no simple sugars. If you have difficulty finding one, you can order my EAT! Formula by calling 1 800 552-1998) As time goes on, you'll find supportive nutrition becomes second nature.

Goal: You will be eating more food and not gaining any fat!

Exercise: Do 12 minutes of aerobic exercise in your target zone every day. Make certain you warm up and cool down gradually

Eat: Lean Protein, Starchy Carb, Fibrous Carb in each meal and attempt to get a Supportive Meal every 3 - 3 1/2 hours

Note: Don't worry if you can't do it perfectly! Simply do better than you're doing now!

A Glance From Day to Day:

Day 1
12 minutes of aerobic exercise in THZ
(Target Heart Zone)

Lean Protein, Starchy Carb, Fibrous Carb
every 3 - 3 1/2 hours

Day 2
12 minutes of aerobic exercise in THZ

Lean Protein, Starchy Carb, Fibrous Carb
every 3 - 3 1/2 hours

Day 3
12 minutes of aerobic exercise in THZ

Lean Protein, Starchy Carb, Fibrous Carb
every 3 - 3 1/2 hours

Days #4 - #6

In these next three days you'll employ Simple Step #6, Challenge and Protect Muscle. You'll begin the metabolism boosting movements with resistance. You'll continue to develop the habit of supportive eating.

Goal: You will begin to stimulate each individual muscle fiber in the body!

Exercise: Perform 1 set of 20 reps of each one of the Standard Exercise Movement with Dumbbells. Follow immediately with your aerobic exercise beginning at 5 minutes and progressing 1 minute each consecutive day

The Standard Exercise Movements
1. Squats
2. Stiff Leg Deadlift
3. Shrug
4. One Arm Row
5. Chest Press
6. Shoulder Press
7. Upright Row
8. Bicep Curl
9. Tricep Extension
10. Standing Calf Raise

Eat: Lean Protein, Starchy Carb, Fibrous Carb in each meal and attempt to get a Supportive Meal every 3 - 3 1/2 hours

A Glance From Day to Day:

Day 4
1 set of 20 reps of each of the Standard
Exercise Movements with dumbbells

5 minutes of aerobic exercise in THZ

Option: 25 abdominal crunches

Day 5
1 set of 20 reps of each of the Standard
Exercise Movements with dumbbells

6 minutes of aerobic exercise in THZ

Option: 25 abdominal crunches

Day 6
1 set of 20 reps of each of the Standard
Exercise Movements with dumbbells

7 minutes of aerobic exercise in THZ

Option: 25 abdominal crunches

Day 7
Rest, Cheat Day

Days #8 - #14

In this second week you'll begin to vary the number of calories you take in from day to day. You'll stimulate greater fat release by alternating a high calorie day (to keep metabolism high) with a high protein low calorie day (A "Protein Day") to accelerate fat release. You'll also progress with the resistance training to stimulate metabolic increase. You'll begin to physiologically initiate some shifts in body composition so your % bodyfat becomes more favorable.

Goal: To incorporate progressive resistance and initiate body composition improvement!

Exercise: You'll perform three sets of each of the Standard Movements. The second set will ask you to use a heavier weight than the first set, and then, with as little rest as comfortable, you'll return to the original weight for the third set. You'll alternate a resistance training day with an aerobc exercise day. You'll begin in Day #9 with 18 minutes in your THZ and add 2 minutes for each successive aerobic session

Eat: Alternate a day in which you have a Lean Protein, Starchy Carb, Fibrous Carb every 3 - 3 1/2 hours with a "Protein Day."

Note: You do not have to do the Protein Days if they become uncomfortable. They do take some getting used to and some people adjust easier than others. Go at your own pace. If you can't get to Protein meals as often as suggested, you might consider a using a protein powder in between meals on the Protein Days.

A Glance From Day to Day:

Day 8
For each of the Standard Exercise Movements,
Perform one set attempting 20 reps, followed by one set
with a heavier weight reaching MMF (Momentary
Muscle Failure) between 8 and 12 reps, then dropping
back to the original weight until again reaching MMF

Protein Day

Day 9
18 minutes of aerobic exercise in THZ

40 abdominal crunches

Lean Protein, Starchy Carb, Fibrous Carb
every 3 - 3 1/2 hours

Day 10
For each of the Standard Exercise Movements,
Perform one set attempting 20 reps, followed by one set
with a heavier weight reaching MMF (Momentary
Muscle Failure) between 8 and 12 reps, then dropping
back to the original weight until again reaching MMF

Protein Day

Day 11
22 minutes of aerobic exercise in THZ

50 abdominal crunches

Lean Protein, Starchy Carb, Fibrous Carb
every 3 - 3 1/2 hours

Day 12
For each of the Standard Exercise Movements,
Perform one set attempting 20 reps, followed by one set
with a heavier weight reaching MMF (Momentary
Muscle Failure) between 8 and 12 reps, then dropping
back to the original weight until again reaching MMF

Protein Day

Day 13
25 minutes of aerobic exercise in THZ

55 abdominal crunches

Lean Protein, Starchy Carb, Fibrous Carb
every 3 - 3 1/2 hours

Day 14
Rest, Cheat Day

Days #15 - #17

In these final three days, you'll increase intensity of resistance training and follow your workouts with aerobic movement. All three of these days will be "Protein Days" to optimize fat release. If, however, it becomes challenging to stay with Protein Days, simply go back to regular Supportive Eating.

Goal: To optimize fat release while maintaining muscle!

Exercise: You'll now incorporate "isolation movements." You'll perform an isolation movement to a point of MMF and immediately move to a compound movement which targets the same muscle or muscle group, again bringing the muscle or muscle group to MMF. You'll repeat each "Superset" three times. Each day will target different muscles using different exercise. You'll follow each workout with a 30-minute aerobic session in your THZ.

Eat: 25% more protein than usual in each meal with a small serving of fibrous carb. Get a "meal" every 3 hours if possible.

A Glance From Day to Day:

Day 15
75 abdominal crunches

Leg Extensions (if you exercise in a gym and are familiar with the machine) or **Lunges** to failure (15-20) immediately followed by **Squats** to failure (15-20)- 3 Supersets

Side Lateral Raise (12-15) immediately followed by **Shoulder Press** to failure (12-15) - 3 supersets

Shrugs (12-15) immediately followed by **Upright Rows** to failure (12-15) - 3 supersets

30 minutes aerobic exercise in THZ

Protein Day

Day 16
78 abdominal crunches

Dumbbell Fly to failure (15-20) immediately followed by **Chest Press** to failure (15-20) - 3 supersets

Bent Over One-Arm Lateral to failure (12-15) immediately followed by **One Arm Row** to failure (12-15) - 3 supersets

Isolation Curl to failure (12-15) immediately followed by **Bicep Curl** to failure (12-15) - 3 supersets

30 minutes aerobic exercise in THZ

Protein Day

Day 17
80 abdominal crunches

Lying Leg Curl to failure (15-20) immediately followed by **Stiff Leg Deadlift** to failure (15-20) - 3 supersets

Seated Calf Raise to failure (15-20) immediately followed by **Standing Calf Raise** to failure (15-20) - 3 supersets

Lying Tricep Extension (12-15) followed by **Dips** to failure (12-15)

30 minutes aerobic exercise in THZ

Protein Day

Follow Day 17 with a high protein high carb day

For the next 3-4 days, simply do what you feel like doing. Then you can return to Day #1.

A Listing of The Exercises

The 10 Standard Exercise Movements
1   Squats
2   Stiff Leg Deadlift
3   Shrug
4   One Arm Row
5   Chest Press
6   Shoulder Press
7   Upright Row
8   Bicep Curl
9   Tricep Extension
10   Standing Calf Raise

Abdominal Movement
11   Abdominal crunches

Supplemental Leg Exercises
12   Lying Leg Curl
13   Lunges
14   Seated Calf Raise

Supplemental Upper Body Exercises
15   Side Lateral Raise
16   Dumbbell Fly
17   Bent Over One-Arm Lateral

Supplemental Arm Movements
18   Lying Tricep Extension
19   Dips
20   Isolation Curl

Following is a very basic outline of each of the movements.
It is simply offered for reference and not intended to act as an
instructional manual. If you are not familiar with the movements,
it is strongly suggested that you meet with a qualified fitness
professional for assistance in form and performance. Performing
resistance movements with incorrect form can result in injury.

The 10 Standard Exercise Movements

1 Squats - Targets the front thighs with assistive involvement from the large hip and gluteal muscles. Stand erect . Slowly bend from knees until thighs are parallel with the ground and slowly return to standing position.

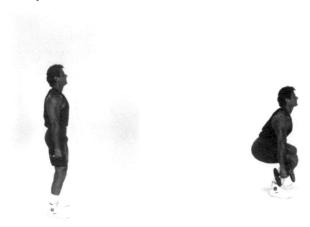

2 Stiff Leg Deadlift - Targets the hamstrings (rear thighs). Stand erect. Keeping legs fixed with very slight bend in knees, bend only from the waist maintaining an arch in the lower back. Bend forward until you feel the rear thigh hamstring muscles stretching and slowly return to erect position.

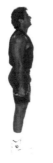
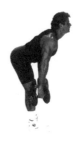

3   **Shrug** - Targets the trapezius of the middle upper back. Hold weights in hands resting on thighs at arms length. Lift shoulders up toward ears and lower. Maintain slight bend in knees throughout.

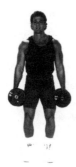 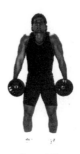

4   **One Arm Row** - Targets the lats, the large muscles at the outside of the upper back. With upper body parallel to the ground, hold weight at arms length. Using the muscles of the upper back, bend elbow until upper arm is adjacent to upper body. Lower.

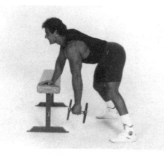 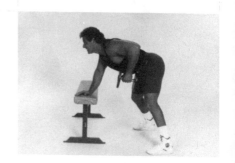

5   Chest Press - Targets the chest muscles with assistance from front shoulders and tricep (rear upper arm). Lying on a bench, or the floor if a bench is not accessible, hold weight in front of you at arms length. Slowly lower to chest and extend.

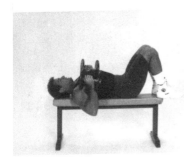
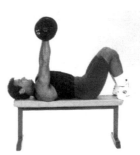

6   Shoulder Press - Targets the shoulders with assistance from triceps. In seated position with back supported, hold weight at arms length overhead. Slowly lower to shoulders and repeat.

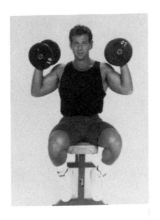
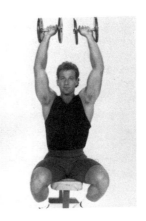

7   **Upright Row** - Targets shoulders and trapezius. Hold weight in front of you resting on front thighs. Bending elbows, pull upward to collarbone and slowly lower. Maintain slight bend in knees throughout.

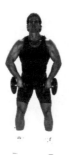
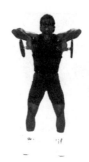

8   **Bicep Curl** - Targets the bicep of the upper arm. Hold weight at arms length resting on thighs. By bending from elbows, use the strength of the bicep muscles to raise arm to shoulders and lower. Maintain slight bend in knees throughout.

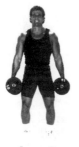
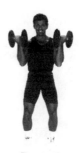

9   Tricep Extension - Targets the triceps (rear upper arm). With upper body parallel to the ground, hold elbow at 90-degree angle so upper arm is adjacent to upper body. Extend the arm and slowly return to starting position.

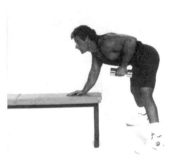 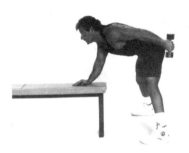

10   Standing Calf Raise - Targets all of the muscles of the calf. With ball of foot on step or platform, lower heel down until you feel a stretch in the calf. Raise all the way up on your toes. Repeat for repetitions. You can hold a dumbbell in one hand for resistance.

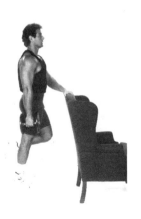 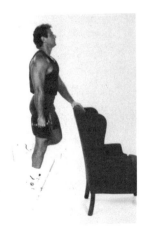

Abdominal Movement

11   Abdominal crunches - Targets the abdominal muscles. Lie on floor with knees bent, feet touching the ground. With hands at ears, elbows out to the sides, raise head and shoulders up toward the ceiling being certain to press your lower back against the ground. Lower and repeat.

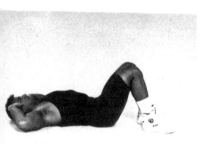 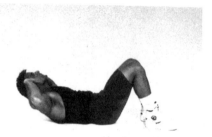

Supplemental Leg Exercises

12   Lying Leg Curl - Targets the hamstring muscles. Lie face down with weight secured safely between feet. Bend from knees until knee joint is at a 90 degree angle and return to starting position.

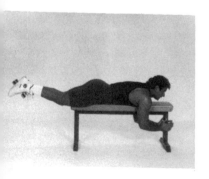 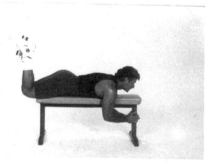

13   Lunges - Targets the front thighs and gluteals. Standing erect, take a step forward with one foot and slowly lower knee of rear leg toward ground. Push off of front leg and return to starting position. Repeat with other leg.

 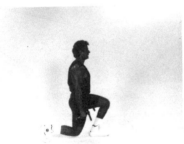

14   Seated Calf Raise - Targets the soleus muscle of the calf. With knees bent at 90 degree angle and balls of feet on step, hold weight on thighs. Lower heels until you feel a stretch of the calf muscle and then raise up on toes.

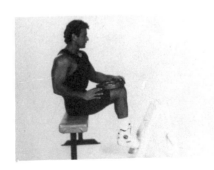 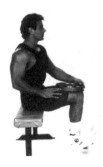

Supplemental Upper Body Exercises

15   **Side Lateral Raise** - Targets the side head of the shoulder muscles. Beginning with arms at sides, raise weights until arms are straight out at sides parallel to the ground and slowly lower. Maintain a bend in knees throughout.

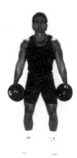 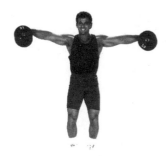

16   **Dumbbell Fly** - Targets and isolates the chest muscles. Lying on back, hold weights are arms length in front of you. Slowly lower the weights out toward the sides and return to starting position.

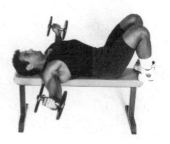 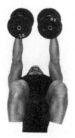

17 **Bent Over One-Arm Lateral** - Targets the rear head of the shoulder which is a visible upper back muscle. With upper body parallel to the ground, hold weight extended toward floor at arms length. Slowly raise out toward the side and slowly return to starting position.

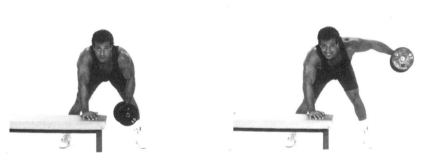

Supplemental Arm Movements
18 **Lying Tricep Extension** - Targets and isolates the triceps. While lying on back, hold weight at arms length in front of you. Slowly bend from elbow keeping elbows pointing up toward the ceiling and then return to starting position.

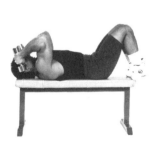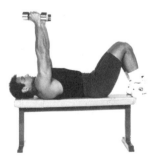

19   Dips - Targets the triceps with assistance from the shoulder and chest muscles. With body being supported at arms length, lower body by bending elbows and return to starting position.

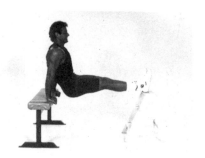 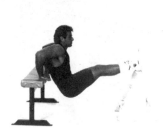

20   Isolation Curl - Targets and isolates the biceps. Rest upper arms against inner thigh. Bend from the elbow raising weight toward shoulder and slowly lower to starting position.

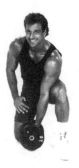 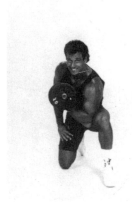

To contact Phil Kaplan's South Florida offices

Phil Kaplan's Fitness, 1304 SW 160th Ave, #337, Ft Lauderdale, FL 33326
Telephone (954) 389-0280   Fax (954) 742-3173
Website: http://philkaplan.com   E-mail: phil@philkaplan.com

<u>Available Through Phil's offices:</u>

* **TRANSFORM!** The book. 368 pages. $39.95

* **EAT! Supportive Nutrition For The Body You Love!** Recipes and detailed tips for making Supportive Nutrition simple. $24.95

* **Mind & Muscle: Fitness For All of You.** 1994   182 pages.

* **Body Transformation Seminar Video.** 2 tapes. 3 hrs. $39.95

* **The Complete Body Transformation Program.** The program that has brought Phil worldwide acclaim. It's all in here! TRANSFORM!, the EAT! recipe book, the Body Transformation seminar video, six audio cassettes, and the complete 17-Week Body Transformation Program with a Journal and Exercise Log. $189.95

* **Resolutions CD.** Copyright 1999. Making your fitness resolution stick! Phil speaks to you and "makes sense." $19.95

* **ENJOY!** Supportive Gourmet Recipes. $19.95

* **EAT! Metabolism Enhancer.** Vanilla or Chocolate. 1 lb. $24.95

* **The Fitness Professional's "Profit 2000" package** featuring Phil's booklet on "influence" in today's confusing fitness market place and 2 hours of audio cassette material teaching fitness professionals to prosper by sharing the true technology of physical change. Learn how to help others get results! $129.00

* **Personal Consultations** with Phil and his staff
* **Seminars** by Phil or select members of his staff

To Order Products call Phil's order line TOLL-FREE:
1 800-552-1998
or use order form on reverse side of this page

ORDER FORM

Fax Orders: (954) 742-3173   **Phone Orders: 1 800 552-1998**
Questions / Phil Kaplan's Offices (954) 389-0280
website: http://philkaplan.com   e-mail: phil@philkaplan.com

To order by mail: Photocopy or tear out this form. Note quantity of each product desired in boxes below, fill in total, enclose check or money order payable to PERSONAL DEVELOPMENT or complete credit card info, and mail to:
Phil Kaplan's Fitness, 1304 SW 160th Ave, #337, Ft Laud, FL 33326

Name _____

Address _____

City, State, Zip _____

Day Phone (   ) _____Home (   ) _____

Fax (   ) _____ E-mail _____

Qty

[   ] **TRANSFORM! The Complete Program.**
    $189.95 + $10 for shipping and handling.

[   ] **EAT! Supportive Nutrition For The Body You Love.**
    $24.95 + $5.00 for shipping and handling.

[   ] **EAT! Metabolism Enhancer** (vanilla)
    $24.95 + $5.00
[   ] **EAT! Metabolism Enhancer** (chocolate)
    $24.95 + $5.00

[   ] **RESOLUTIONS CD**
    $19.95 + $5.00

Order Total $_____

Other Products

Qty	Item	Price	Ship	Total
___	_____	___	___	___
___	_____	___	___	___
___	_____	___	___	___

[ ] MasterCard   [ ] Visa   [ ] AMEX   [ ] Discover
Acct # _____Exp _____
        Signature _____

All Prices are in U.S. Dollars. In Florida add 6% sales tax.